HANDBOOK OF MEDICAL BIOCHEMISTRY
VOLUME 1

FOUNDATIONS OF MOLECULAR AND METABOLIC MEDICINE

Prof. Ramesh Chandra
and Dr. Heerak Chugh

ALLIED HEALTH PRESS

Handbook of Medical Biochemistry Volume 1

Foundations of Molecular and Metabolic Medicine

Authors: **Prof. Ramesh Chandra and Dr. Heerak Chugh**

Allied Health Press
4164 Lakeshore Road
Burlington ON L7L 1A4
Canada
www.alliedhealthpress.com
Email: orders@arclereducation.com

ISBN: 978-1-77956-814-4

ABOUT THE AUTHORS

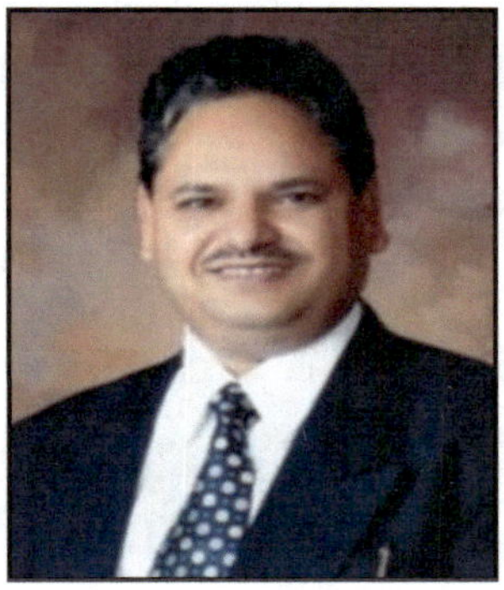

Prof. Ramesh Chandra is a distinguished scientist; Fellow of the Royal Society of Chemistry, London and an outstanding researcher in the field of Biomedical Sciences. Currently, he is the Vice-Chancellor at Maharaja Surajmal Brij University, Bharatpur, Rajasthan, and Founder Director of Dr. B. R. Ambedkar Center for Biomedical Research (ACBR), University of Delhi. He is Official resource person to the Minister and Department of Science and Technology in the kingdom of Lesotho, South Africa.

He started his research career at the University of Delhi, then at The New York Hospital-Cornell University Medical College, and The Rockefeller University, New York; State University of New York at Stonybrook, Harvard University Medical School-Massachusetts General Hospital (MGH) jointly at MIT, Cambridge, USA.

Prof. Chandra has been Vice-Chancellor, Bundelkhand University, Jhansi (1999-2005) as well as President of the Indian Chemical Society, Member, Planning Commission, Government of U.P. India; Secretary - Zaheer Science Foundation, New Delhi and Non-Official Director, Rashtriya Ispat Nigam Ltd, Government of India. He was also Head of the Department of Chemistry, University of Delhi.

He is recipient of several international recognitions: J. William Fulbright Scholarship, The Rockefeller Foundation USA-Biotechnology Career Award, Award of the Highest Honor of Soka University, Tokyo, Japan; Millennium Plaques of Honor (Life Time Achievement Award for contribution in Science & Technology) by the Indian Science Congress Association (ISCA), Lifetime Achievement Award of the Indian Chemical Society (1CS); UGC Research Scientist Award; UGC Career Award; Rajib Goyal Award for Young Scientists and others.

Prof. Chandra shows deep commitment to the cause of higher education & research and possesses in ample measure quality of dynamic leadership, vision required for building academic institutions and excelled in his academic pursuits. To illustrate, he has to his credit several international patents, 9 Books; 28 Book Chapters; and more than 400 original Scientific Research Papers in International journals of repute. He has mentored more than 100 Ph.D. students.

In recognition of his outstanding Scientific Research and Administrative Qualities, Prof Ramesh Chandra has been conferred Capital Foundation Dr A.P.J. Abdul Kalam National Award.

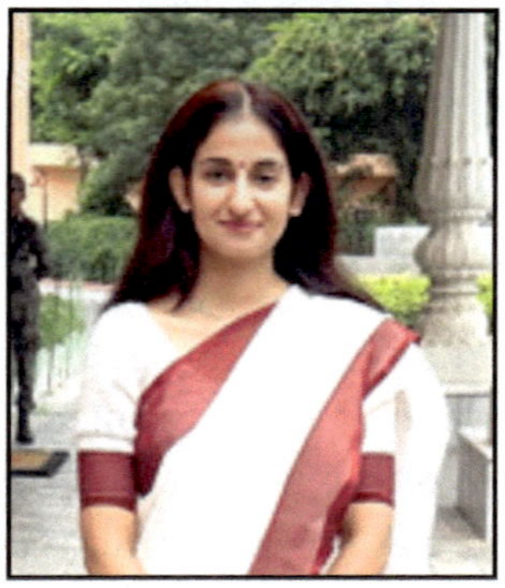

Dr Heerak Chugh is a life scientist who is currently working as a Senior Researcher funded by Indian Council of Medical Research (ICMR) at University of Delhi, Delhi. She is also teaching as an Adjunct Assistant Professor at Maharaja Surajmal Brij University, Rajasthan.

Her Research focusses on advancing our current understanding of cancer and exploring therapeutic interventions to improve treatment (patient) outcomes. She has extensive experience in Cell biology, molecular biology, biochemistry, cancer biology, chemical biology, biophysical chemistry, chemotherapeutics, drug delivery and cancer nanomedicine.

Dr Heerak Chugh completed her graduation and postgraduation in Life Science from Sri Venkateswara, University of Delhi, Delhi and Central University of Punjab, Bathinda, Punjab, respectively.

Dr Heerak Chugh developed her research interest while working as a research intern at CSIR-IGIB where she was working on synthesizing plant-based nanoparticles and cationic nanoparticles as novel anti-microbial agents. To continue her research interests, Dr Heerak Chugh joined a Ph.D. programme in University of Delhi, Drug Discovery and Development Laboratory, Department of Chemistry, University of Delhi wherein she worked on increasing the therapeutic efficacy of Noscapine, an anti-cancer agent.

Dr Chugh was awarded prestigious Prime Minister Fellowship for Doctoral Research by Science and Engineering Research Board (SERB), Government of India and Confederation of Indian Industry (CII); until now, she is the only recipient from University of Delhi. She was also awarded Junior Research Fellowship through National Eligibility Test (All India Rank 60). Further, she was also awarded Senior Research Fellowship by Indian Council of Medical Research.

During her Ph.D., she worked at Department of Biological Sciences, Purdue University, Indiana, USA as Science and Engineering Research Board, Government of India funded Overseas Doctoral Visiting Fellow where she studied HYPE protein and its role in cancer.

She was one of the subject matter experts on Voet's Biochemistry Adapted Edition 2021. She has published over a dozen research articles in various peer-reviewed International Journals, and continues to work and publish actively in the field of cancer biology and cancer therapeutics. She also serves as an invited reviewer for various international journals.

Brief Table of Contents

1. Introduction to Medical Biochemistry	1
2. Biomolecules	35
3. Enzymes	69
4. Bioenergetics	103
5. Carbohydrate Metabolism	135
6. Lipid Metabolism	171
7. Protein and Amino Acid Metabolism	207
8. Nucleotide Metabolism	245
9. Vitamins and Coenzymes	281
10. Hormones and Signal Transduction	309
11. Molecular Biology	343
12. Genetic Disorders	377
Index	403

Getting Started with This Book

Chapter Openers

A list of Chapter Outline is presented providing a brief Introduction to what will be covered in the chapter.

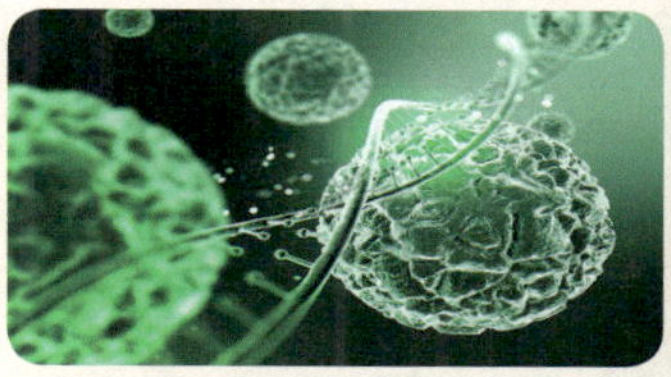

Introduction

Often referred to as the science of life, biology is a broad field of study aimed at comprehending the several kinds of life on Earth, from tiny creatures to sophisticated multicellular entities. Comprising several subfields, including molecular biology, ecology, and evolutionary biology, each of which advances our knowledge of living systems, this field clarifies the mechanisms controlling life events, including development, reproduction, and interaction with the surroundings, which is the central goal of biology. Moreover, biology fills in the void between the natural sciences and medicine by offering a necessary understanding of health, illness, and the interactions between organisms and their environments. Dealing with urgent global issues such as climate change, biodiversity loss, and new diseases depends on an awareness of these complex biological interactions, therefore highlighting the critical part biology plays in modern civilization. Fundamentally, biology explores and tests ideas about the living world using the scientific method. Through methodical observation and experimentation,

LEARNING OBJECTIVES

After studying this chapter, you will be able to:

1. Discuss the scientific method in biology;
2. Explain the cell theory;
3. Discuss the genetics and heredity;
4. Evolution and natural selection;
5. Focus on ecology and ecosystems;
6. Learn about human biology;
7. Evaluate the plant biology;
8. Explain the microbiology;
9. Focus on current trends in biology.

1.1. The Scientific Method in Biology

Learning Outcome

1. Describe the steps of the scientific method;
2. Focus on hypothesis formation;
3. Learn about experimental design.

Learning Outcomes

The beginning of each section of every chapter contains a set of Learning Outcomes that inform students of concepts they should understand. These outcomes help students understand what they should be able to do if they have mastered the material in that section.

Test Your Knowledge

Throughout each chapter, Test Your Knowledge cues you to note which topics have been covered and to self-test your understanding of the material presented.

Test Your Knowledge

1. Explain why correlation does not imply causation in scientific experiments.
2. How does the scientific method help reduce the influence of personal opinions in research?

Chapter Summary

The Summary Section appear at the end of each chapter and summarize main concepts covered throughout the chapter. These points provide key concepts in an engaging and meaningful way.

Summary

The investigation of biological principles highlights the importance of a comprehensive view of life by reflecting the intricate interactions that occur within living systems. The complexity of biology goes beyond individual species or systems, as this essay highlights; it also includes the interactions that mold ecosystems and affect biodiversity. Researchers can conduct in-depth analyses of metabolomic data using sophisticated technologies like MetaboAnalyst, which offer insights into the molecular mechanisms underlying these interactions. As demonstrated by the developments in MetaboAnalyst, for example, the integration of diverse omics data promotes a thorough understanding of metabolic pathways and helps identify important biological markers necessary for research on development and disease (Chong et al., 2018). Additionally, the phenomenon of ecological invasions is a key component of biological research and a vital field of study. The introduction of non-native species into unfamiliar habitats has significant ramifications and calls for multidisciplinary management strategies. Examining the origins and effects of these biological incursions, invasion science has become a crucial field that highlights the need to comprehend ecological dynamics and community interactions. As interest in biological invasions increases, new findings are emerging that put conventional ecological theories and practices to the test. The importance of incorporating various scientific viewpoints is shown by this developing discipline, which also highlights how invasive species shape ecosystems and advances our knowledge of ecological resilience (David et al., 2013). When taken as a whole, these discoveries from invasion science and metabolomics highlight the value of multidisciplinary biology research. Fostering cross-disciplinary collaboration and utilizing technological breakthroughs to improve our comprehension of intricate biological interactions are crucial as we look to the future of biological research. In addition to deepening our understanding of the complexities of life, this method lays the groundwork for tackling urgent environmental issues. Future studies can ensure the continued relevance of biology in a world that is constantly changing by acknowledging the interconnection of biological systems and opening the door to creative solutions that support sustainability and biodiversity conservation. We might imagine a thorough comprehension of life that serves both academia and society at large through ongoing investigation and integration of scientific knowledge.

Knowledge Assessment

The chapter includes material designed to review and reinforce each content. It includes Critical Thinking Questions to help test of your understanding of information presented in the chapter and Short answer Questions to review your understanding of the key concepts presented in the chapter.

Critical Thinking Questions

1. **Who is known as the "Father of Modern Biology"?**
   a. Aristotle
   b. Charles Darwin
   c. Gregor Mendel
   d. Louis Pasteur
2. **What is the basic unit of life?**
   a. Atom
   b. Molecule
   c. Cell
   d. Organism
3. **Which branch of biology studies the interaction of organisms with their environment?**
   a. Genetics
   b. Ecology
   c. Physiology
   d. Botany
4. **Which macromolecule is the main source of energy for living organisms?**
   a. Proteins
   b. Lipids
   c. Carbohydrates
   d. Nucleic acids
5. **DNA is primarily responsible for which function in living organisms?**
   a. Energy production
   b. Protein synthesis
   c. Storing genetic information
   d. Regulating body temperature

Short Answer Questions

1. What is biology, and why is it important to study biology?
2. What are the three main domains of life, and how are they different from one another?
3. Define homeostasis and give an example of how it works in living organisms.
4. What is the cell theory, and why is it fundamental to biology?
5. How do autotrophs and heterotrophs differ in the way they obtain energy?
6. What is the scientific method, and how is it applied in biological research?
7. Discuss how biology helps address global challenges such as climate change, disease, and food security.
8. Explain the levels of biological organization from the smallest unit to the largest. Provide examples at each level.
9. Describe the relationship between structure and function in biology, giving specific examples from cells or organs.
10. How has the discovery of genetics shaped our understanding of inheritance and variation among organisms?

Supplementary Materials

Key Terms: A list of key terms is given for quick reference

KEY TERMS FROM THIS CHAPTER

Annotation enrichment analysis	Biological structure	Cell
Cell theory	Cellular structure	Ecology
Ecosystems	Genetics	Human biology
Microbiology	Natural selection	Organism
Plant biology		

Further Resources: Recommendations for additional readings, websites, and multimedia resources.

References

1. Argelaguet, R., Velten, B., Arnol, D., Dietrich, S., Zenz, T., Marioni, J. C., Buettner, F., et al. (2018). Multi-omics factor analysis—A framework for unsupervised integration of multi-omics data sets. *Molecular Systems Biology, 14*. https://doi.org/10.15252/msb.20178124.
2. Bacher, S., Blackburn, T. M., Essl, F., & Genovesi, P. (2017). *Socio-Economic Impact Classification of Alien Taxa (SEICAT).* https://core.ac.uk/download/286567949.pdf (accessed on 8th March 2025).
3. Barnett, R., Brace, S., Cucchi, T., & Dobney, K. (2013). *Divergent Evolutionary Processes Associated with Colonization of Offshore Islands.* https://core.ac.uk/download/20664364.pdf (accessed on 8th March 2025).

Detailed Table of Contents

List of Figures xv
Preface xxv

CHAPTER 1

Introduction to Medical Biochemistry 1

Introduction 1
1.1. Biomolecules in Medicine 5
1.1.1. Structure and Function of Proteins 5
1.1.2. Role of Carbohydrates in Health and Disease 6
1.1.3. Significance of Lipids and Nucleic Acids 7
1.2. Metabolic Pathways 8
1.2.1. Overview of Catabolic and Anabolic Pathways 9
1.2.2. Key Metabolic Pathways in Human Health 10
1.2.3. Regulation of Metabolism and Its Clinical Implications 11
1.3. Enzymes and Enzyme Kinetics 12
1.3.1. Enzyme Structure and Function 13
1.3.2. Factors Affecting Enzyme Activity 14
1.3.3. Clinical Significance of Enzyme Assays 15
1.4. Genetic Biochemistry 16
1.4.1. DNA Structure and Replication 16
1.4.2. RNA Synthesis and Protein Translation 18
1.4.3. Genetic Mutations and Their Biochemical Consequences 18
1.5. Hormones and Signaling Molecules 20
1.5.1. Types of Hormones and Their Functions 20
1.5.2. Mechanisms of Hormone Action 21
1.5.3. Hormonal Imbalances and Related Diseases 22
1.6. Clinical Applications of Medical Biochemistry 24
1.6.1. Diagnostic Techniques in Biochemistry 24
1.6.2. Biochemical Markers in Disease Management 25
1.6.3. Therapeutic Interventions Based on Biochemical Principles 26
Summary 28
References 31

CHAPTER 2

Biomolecules 35

Introduction 35
2.1. Carbohydrates 39
2.1.1. Structure and Classification 39
2.1.2. Functions in Living Organisms 40
2.1.3. Examples of Carbohydrates in Nature 41
2.2. Proteins 42
2.2.1. Amino Acids and Protein Structure 43
2.2.2. Role of Proteins in Cellular Functions 44
2.2.3. Enzymes as Biological Catalysts 45
2.3. Lipids 46
2.3.1. Types of Lipids and Their Structures 46
2.3.2. Functions of Lipids in the Body 47
2.3.3. Lipids in Energy Storage and Membrane Formation 48
2.4. Nucleic Acids 49
2.4.1. Structure of DNA and RNA 50

2.4.2. Role of Nucleic Acids in Heredity 51
2.4.3. Importance of Nucleotides in Metabolism 52
2.5. Metabolism of Biomolecules 54
2.5.1. Catabolism and Anabolism 55
2.5.2. Energy Production from Biomolecules 56
2.5.3. Regulation of Metabolic Pathways 57
2.6. Biomolecules in Health and Disease 58
2.6.1. Role of Biomolecules in Nutrition 59
2.6.2. Biomolecules and Their Link to Diseases 60
2.6.3. Therapeutic Applications of Biomolecules 60
Summary 62
References 65

CHAPTER 3

Enzymes 69

Introduction 69
3.1. Structure of Enzymes 72
3.1.1. Basic Components of Enzymes 73
3.1.2. The Role of Active Sites 74
3.1.3. Enzyme Specificity and Substrate Interaction 75
3.2. Mechanism of Enzyme Action 76
3.2.1. The Lock and Key Model 76
3.2.2. The Induced Fit Model 77
3.2.3. Factors Affecting Enzyme Activity 78
3.3. Types of Enzymes 80
3.3.1. Classification Based on Function 81
3.3.2. Enzymes in Metabolic Pathways 81
3.3.3. Industrial Enzymes and Their Applications 82
Test Your Knowledge 83
3.4.1. Understanding Reaction Rates 84
3.4.2. Michaelis–Menten Kinetics 84
3.4.3. Enzyme Inhibitors and Activators 85
3.5. Enzymes in Human Health 87
3.5.1. Role of Enzymes in Digestion 88
3.5.2. Enzymes in Disease Diagnosis 89
3.5.3. Therapeutic Enzymes and Treatments 90
3.6. Environmental Impact of Enzymes 91
3.6.1. Enzymes in Bioremediation 92
3.6.2. Role of Enzymes in Agriculture 92
3.6.3. Enzymes and Sustainability 93
Summary 95
References 98

CHAPTER 4

Bioenergetics 103

Introduction 103
4.1. Fundamental Concepts of Energy in Biology 106
4.1.1. Types of Energy Relevant to Biological Processes 107
4.1.2. Laws of Thermodynamics and Their Application 108
4.1.3. Energy Transformations in Living Organisms 109
4.2. Cellular Respiration 110
4.2.1. Overview of Aerobic and Anaerobic Respiration 111
4.2.2. Key Metabolic Pathways Involved 112
4.2.3. Role of ATP in Energy Transfer 112
4.3. Photosynthesis 114
4.3.1. Process of Converting Light Energy into Chemical Energy 114
4.3.2. Importance of Chlorophyll and Light-Dependent Reactions 115
4.3.3. Calvin Cycle and the Synthesis of Glucose 116
4.4. Bioenergetics in Muscle Function 118
4.4.1. Energy Requirements During Muscle Contraction 118
4.4.2. Role of Creatine Phosphate and Glycolysis 119
4.4.3. Impact of Aerobic vs. Anaerobic Metabolism on Performance 120
4.5. Bioenergetics and Metabolism 121
4.5.1. Catabolic vs. Anabolic Pathways 122
4.5.2. Regulation of Metabolic Pathways 123
4.5.3. Role of Enzymes in Bioenergetic Processes 124
4.6. Applications of Bioenergetics 125
4.6.1. Bioenergetics in Medicine and Health 126
4.6.2. Environmental Implications and Bioenergetics 127
4.6.3. Future Research Directions in Bioenergetics 127
Summary 129
References 132

CHAPTER 5

Carbohydrate Metabolism 135

Introduction 135

5.1. Types of Carbohydrates 139

5.1.1. Simple Carbohydrates 140

5.1.2. Complex Carbohydrates 141

5.1.3. Dietary Fiber 142

5.2. Digestion of Carbohydrates 143

5.2.1. Role of Salivary Amylase 144

5.2.2. Enzymatic Breakdown in the Small Intestine 144

5.2.3. Absorption of Monosaccharides 145

5.3. Glycolysis 147

5.3.1. Overview of the Glycolytic Pathway 148

5.3.2. Energy Yield from Glycolysis 148

5.3.3. Regulation of Glycolysis 150

Test Your Knowledge 151

5.4.1. Definition and Purpose of Gluconeogenesis 152

5.4.2. Key Enzymes Involved 154

5.4.3. Differences Between Glycolysis and Gluconeogenesis 154

5.5. Glycogen Metabolism 156

5.5.1. Glycogenesis: Formation of Glycogen 156

5.5.2. Glycogenolysis: Breakdown of Glycogen 157

5.5.3. Hormonal Regulation of Glycogen Metabolism 158

5.6. Role of Insulin and Glucagon 159

5.6.1. Insulin's Effect on Carbohydrate Metabolism 160

5.6.2. Glucagon's Role in Energy Mobilization 161

5.6.3. Interaction Between Insulin and Glucagon 162

Summary 163

References 166

CHAPTER 6

Lipid Metabolism 171

Introduction 171

6.1. Types of Lipids 174

6.1.1. Fatty Acids 175

6.1.2. Triglycerides (TGs) 176

6.1.3. Phospholipids 177

6.2. Digestion and Absorption of Lipids 178

6.2.1. Role of Bile Salts 180

6.2.2. Enzymatic Breakdown by Lipases 181

6.2.3. Absorption in the Intestinal Mucosa 181

6.3. Transport of Lipids in the Body 183

6.3.1. Chylomicrons and Lipoproteins 184

6.3.2. Role of the Lymphatic System 185

6.3.3. Lipid Transport in the Bloodstream 186

6.4. Beta-Oxidation of Fatty Acids 187

6.4.1. Process of Fatty Acid Activation 188

6.4.2. Mitochondrial Transport of Fatty Acids 189

6.4.3. Energy Production from Beta-Oxidation 190

6.5. Lipogenesis 191

6.5.1. Conversion of Excess Carbohydrates to Fat 192

6.5.2. Role of Acetyl-CoA in Lipogenesis 193

6.5.3. Regulation of Lipogenesis by Hormones 193

6.6. Disorders Related to Lipid Metabolism 195

6.6.1. Hyperlipidemia 196

6.6.2. Fatty Liver Disease 196

6.6.3. Metabolic Syndrome (MS) 197

Summary 199

References 202

CHAPTER 7

Protein and Amino Acid Metabolism 207

Introduction 207

7.1. Structure of Proteins 211

7.1.1. Amino Acid Composition and Structure 212

7.1.2. Levels of Protein Structure: Primary, Secondary, Tertiary, and Quaternary 213

7.1.3. Role of Protein Folding in Function 214

7.2. Digestion of Proteins 215

7.2.1. Process of Protein Digestion in the Gastrointestinal Tract 216

7.2.2. Enzymes Involved in Protein Breakdown 217

7.2.3. Absorption of Amino Acids in the Small Intestine 218

7.3. Amino Acid Metabolism 219

7.3.1. Transamination and Deamination Processes 220
7.3.2. Role of Amino Acids in Energy Production 221
7.3.3. Synthesis of Non-Essential Amino Acids 223
7.4. Protein Synthesis **224**
7.4.1. Overview of Transcription and Translation 224
7.4.2. Role of Ribosomes in Protein Synthesis 226
7.4.3. Post-Translational Modifications of Proteins 227
7.5. Regulation of Protein Metabolism **229**
7.5.1. Hormonal Regulation of Protein Synthesis and Degradation 229
7.5.2. Nutritional Factors Affecting Protein Metabolism 231
7.5.3. Impact of Exercise on Protein Metabolism 231
7.6. Disorders Related to Protein Metabolism **233**
7.6.1. Inborn Errors of Metabolism (e.g., Phenylketonuria) 233
7.6.2. Protein-Energy Malnutrition (e.g., Kwashiorkor and Marasmus) 234
7.6.3. Effects of Excessive Protein Intake 236
Summary **237**
References **240**

CHAPTER 8

Nucleotide Metabolism 245

Introduction **245**
8.1. Structure of Nucleotides **248**
8.1.1. Components of Nucleotides: Nitrogenous Bases, Sugars, and Phosphate Groups 249
8.1.2. Differences Between DNA and RNA Nucleotides 250
8.1.3. Role of Nucleotide Structure in Metabolism 251
8.2. Nucleotide Synthesis Pathways **252**
8.2.1. De Novo Synthesis Pathway 253
8.2.2. Salvage Pathway 254
8.2.3. Regulation of Nucleotide Synthesis 255
8.3. Purine Metabolism **256**
8.3.1. Synthesis of Purine Nucleotides 257
8.3.2. Degradation of Purines and Uric Acid Formation 258
8.3.3. Disorders Related to Purine Metabolism 259
8.4. Pyrimidine Metabolism **261**
8.4.1. Synthesis of Pyrimidine Nucleotides 262
8.4.2. Degradation of Pyrimidines 263
8.4.3. Clinical Implications of Pyrimidine Metabolism Disorders 264
8.5. Nucleotide Interconversion **266**
8.5.1. Role of Nucleoside Diphosphate Kinases (NDPKs) 266
8.5.2. Importance of Nucleotide Triphosphate Interconversion 267
8.5.3. Impact on Energy Metabolism and Signaling 268
8.6. Nucleotide Metabolism and Disease **269**
8.6.1. Cancer and Altered Nucleotide Metabolism 270
8.6.2. Genetic Disorders Affecting Nucleotide Metabolism 271
8.6.3. Therapeutic Targets in Nucleotide Metabolism 272
Summary **274**
References **277**

CHAPTER 9

Vitamins and Coenzymes 281

Introduction **281**
9.1. Types of Vitamins **285**
9.1.1. Water-Soluble Vitamins 285
9.1.2. Fat-Soluble Vitamins 286
9.1.3. Role of Vitamins in Human Health 287
9.2. Functions of Coenzymes **289**
9.2.1. Role in Enzymatic Reactions 289
9.2.2. Examples of Common Coenzymes 290
9.2.3. Importance of Coenzymes in Metabolism 291
9.3. Sources of Vitamins **292**
9.3.1. Dietary Sources of Vitamins 293
9.3.2. Supplementation Options 293
9.3.3. Recommended Daily Allowances 294
9.4. Deficiency and Excess of Vitamins **295**
9.4.1. Consequences of Vitamin Deficiency 296
9.4.2. Symptoms of Vitamin Excess 297
9.4.3. Public Health Implications 298
9.5. Research and Advances in Vitamin and Coenzyme Studies **300**

9.5.1. Recent Findings in Vitamin Research 300
9.5.2. Innovations in Coenzyme Applications 301
9.5.3. Future Directions in Nutritional Science 302
Summary 304
References 307

CHAPTER 10

Hormones and Signal Transduction 309

Introduction 309
10.1. Types of Hormones 312
10.1.1. Peptide Hormones 313
10.1.2. Steroid Hormones 314
10.1.3. Amine Hormones 315
10.2. Mechanisms of Hormone Action 316
10.2.1. Receptor Binding 317
10.2.2. Intracellular Signaling Pathways 318
10.2.3. Gene Expression Modulation 318
10.3. Signal Transduction Pathways 319
10.3.1. G-Protein Coupled Receptors (GPCRs) 320
10.3.2. Receptor Tyrosine Kinases (RTKs) 321
10.3.3. Ion Channel Receptors 322
10.4. Hormonal Regulation of Metabolism 324
10.4.1. Insulin and Glucose Metabolism 324
10.4.2. Glucagon and Energy Mobilization 325
10.4.3. Thyroid Hormones and Metabolic Rate 326
10.5. Hormones and Homeostasis 327
10.5.1. Role of Hormones in Maintaining Blood Pressure 328
10.5.2. Hormonal Control of Water Balance 329
10.5.3. Regulation of Calcium Levels 330
10.6. Disorders Related to Hormonal Imbalance 331
10.6.1. Diabetes Mellitus 332
10.6.2. Hyperthyroidism and Hypothyroidism 333
10.6.3. Cushing's Syndrome 334
Summary 336
References 339

CHAPTER 11

Molecular Biology 343

Introduction 343
11.1. Structure of DNA 346
11.1.1. Double Helix Model and Its Significance 346
11.1.2. Nucleotide Composition and Base Pairing 347
11.1.3. Chromatin Structure and Organization 348
11.2. DNA Replication 350
11.2.1. Mechanisms of DNA Replication 351
11.2.2. Role of Enzymes in Replication 352
11.2.3. Importance of Fidelity and Error Correction 353
11.3. Gene Expression 354
11.3.1. Transcription Process and Regulation 354
11.3.2. Translation and the Role of Ribosomes 355
11.3.3. Post-Transcriptional Modifications 356
11.4. Molecular Techniques 357
11.4.1. Polymerase Chain Reaction (PCR) 358
11.4.2. Gel Electrophoresis and Its Applications 359
11.4.3. CRISPR-Cas9 Technology and Gene Editing 360
11.5. Protein Structure and Function 362
11.5.1. Levels of Protein Structure: Primary to Quaternary 363
11.5.2. Enzyme Function and Kinetics 363
11.5.3. Role of Proteins in Cellular Processes 364
11.6. Applications of Molecular Biology 365
11.6.1. Biotechnology and Genetic Engineering 366
11.6.2. Medical Applications and Personalized Medicine 366
11.6.3. Environmental and Agricultural Advancements 367
Summary 369
References 372

CHAPTER 12

Genetic Disorders 377

Introduction 377
12.1. Types of Genetic Disorders 380
12.1.1. Single-Gene Disorders 380

12.1.2. Chromosomal Disorders 381
12.1.3. Multifactorial Disorders 382
12.2. Causes of Genetic Disorders 384
12.2.1. Mutations in DNA 384
12.2.2. Inheritance Patterns 385
12.2.3. Environmental Factors 386
12.3. Symptoms and Diagnosis 387
12.3.1. Common Symptoms of Genetic Disorders 388
12.3.2. Diagnostic Techniques 389
12.3.3. Role of Genetic Counseling 390
12.4. Treatment Options 392
12.4.1. Medical Management 392
12.4.2. Gene Therapy 393
12.4.3. Lifestyle and Supportive Care 394
Summary 396
References 399

Index 403

LIST OF FIGURES

Figure 1.1. Medical biochemistry

Figure 1.2. Laboratory scientist handling blood samples in a biosafety cabinet

Figure 1.3. James Watson and Francis Crick with their DNA model at the Cavendish Laboratories in 1953

Figure 1.4. 3D illustration of a DNA double helix structure with surrounding molecules

Figure 1.5. Protein structure and function

Figure 1.6. The role of carbohydrate in health and disease

Figure 1.7. Metabolic pathways

Figure 1.8. Anabolic pathways are those that require energy to synthesize larger molecules. Catabolic pathways are those that generate energy by breaking down larger molecules. Both types of pathways are required for maintaining the cell's energy balance

Figure 1.9. Illustration of obesity-related health risks and medical consultation

Figure 1.10. Michaelis–Menten saturation curve of an enzyme reaction. Parameter values used are V_{max} = 3.4 and K_m = 1.7

Figure 1.11. (a) According to the lock-and-key model, the shape of an enzyme's active site is a perfect fit for the substrate. (b) According to the induced fit model, the active site is somewhat flexible and can change shape in order to bond with the substrate

Figure 1.12. Factors affecting enzyme activity

Figure 1.13. Illustration of a scientist analyzing genetic data and DNA sequencing

Figure 1.14. DNA replication. During the process of DNA replication, the original DNA molecule is uncoiled by DNA helicase, separating the two strands. Each then forms the template upon which DNA polymerase synthesizes a new double helix, with complementary nucleotide pairs ensuring faithful replication of the original DNA sequence

Figure 1.15. Colored 3D representation of a DNA double helix strand

Figure 1.16. Types of hormones

Figure 1.17. Mechanism of steroid hormone action

Figure 1.18. Hormonal imbalance

Figure 1.19. Serological tests

Figure 1.20. Gloved hand handling microcentrifuge tubes for PCR analysis

Figure 2.1. Biomolecules

Figure 2.2. Definition of biomolecules

Figure 2.3. Types of biomolecules

Figure 2.4. Carbohydrates
Figure 2.5. Classification of carbohydrates
Figure 2.6. Examples of carbohydrates
Figure 2.7. Protein
Figure 2.8. Amino acids
Figure 2.9. Molecular model of a hemoglobin protein structure
Figure 2.10. Lipids
Figure 2.11. Lipids are useful chemical compounds in all of your body's cells
Figure 2.12. Functions of lipids
Figure 2.13. Nucleic acids
Figure 2.14. Structure of DNA and RNA
Figure 2.15. Nucleotide
Figure 2.16. Different types of biochemicals that are involved in various metabolic processes of a living cell and organism
Figure 2.17. Catabolism and anabolism
Figure 2.18. Glucose is one of the most abundant carbohydrates. Cells can use glucose for immediate energy or store glucose for later use as a polysaccharide, such as starch. In addition, cells use glucose to build various organic molecules
Figure 2.19. Graphic representation of biomolecules surrounded by virus-like particles
Figure 2.20. Role of biomolecules in nutrition
Figure 3.1. Enzymes
Figure 3.2. Enzymes in the body
Figure 3.3. Structure of enzymes
Figure 3.4. Enzymes are proteins
Figure 3.5. Active site of an enzyme
Figure 3.6. Enzyme specificity
Figure 3.7. Mechanism of enzyme action, describes how the substrate reacts with the enzyme, which results in the formation of the enzyme-substrate complex finally, this complex is converted into products and leaves the enzyme without any changes
Figure 3.8. Lock and key model
Figure 3.9. Induced fit model of enzymes
Figure 3.10. Factors affecting enzyme activity
Figure 3.11. Types of enzymes
Figure 3.12. Control of metabolic pathways using enzymes
Figure 3.13. Enzyme kinetics
Figure 3.14. Curve of the Michaelis–Menten equation labelled in accordance with IUBMB recommendations
Figure 3.15. Allosteric inhibition works by indirectly inducing a conformational change to the active

site such that the substrate no longer fits. In contrast, in allosteric activation, the activator molecule modifies the shape of the active site to allow a better fit of the substrate

Figure 3.16. A diagram showing the three main enzymes involved in digestion, breaking down three large polymers into their monomer subunits

Figure 3.17. A diagram showing the main organs of the human digestive system, with the sites of production (shown by circles) and action (shown by crosses) of amylases in green, those of proteases in pink, and those of lipases in orange

Figure 3.18. Enzymes for disease diagnosis

Figure 3.19. Therapeutic enzymes are used in the treatment of a variety of disorders and diseases

Figure 3.20. Application of enzymes in bioremediation of solid wastes and soils

Figure 3.21. Enzymes used in agriculture

Figure 4.1. Bioenergetics

Figure 4.2. Artistic representation of neural activity and bioenergetic signaling in the brain

Figure 4.3. Energy and metabolism

Figure 4.4. Types of energy

Figure 4.5. Laws of thermodynamics

Figure 4.6. Cellular respiration

Figure 4.7. Anaerobic respiration

Figure 4.8. ATP hydrolysis. The high-energy bonds of ATP can be broken through the addition of water, which releases high amounts of energy in addition to ADP and an inorganic phosphate

Figure 4.9. Photosynthesis

Figure 4.10. Converting light energy to chemical energy

Figure 4.11. The light-dependent reactions

Figure 4.12. Overview of the Calvin cycle pathway

Figure 4.13. Bioenergetics in muscle function

Figure 4.14. A simplified diagram showing the role of creatine phosphate in transporting energy for muscle contraction

Figure 4.15. Aerobic and anaerobic exercise

Figure 4.16. Bioenergetics and metabolism

Figure 4.17. The view of microbial metabolism as a thermodynamic energy converter. Catabolic reactions have a large negative free energy gradient, driving anabolic reactions

Figure 4.18. Bioenergetics of the electron transport chain and the TCA/Krebs cycle

Figure 4.19. Physician consulting with an elderly patient in a clinical setting

Figure 4.20. Conceptual illustration of human bioenergetics and molecular pathways

Figure 5.1. Overview of carbohydrate metabolism

Figure 5.2. Importance of carbohydrates in human nutrition

Figure 5.3. Types of carbohydrates

Figure 5.4. Foods containing simple sugars

Figure 5.5. Complex carbohydrates

Figure 5.6. Variety of fiber-rich foods including fruits, vegetables, legumes, and grains

Figure 5.7. The digestive system

Figure 5.8. The enzyme salivary amylase breaks starch into smaller polysaccharides and maltose

Figure 5.9. Digestion and absorption of carbohydrates in the small intestine

Figure 5.10. Carbohydrate uptake and absorption

Figure 5.11. During the energy-consuming phase of glycolysis, two ATPs are consumed, transferring two phosphates to the glucose molecule. The glucose molecule then splits into two three-carbon compounds, each containing a phosphate. During the second phase, an additional phosphate is added to each of the three-carbon compounds. The energy for this endergonic reaction is provided by the removal (oxidation) of two electrons from each three-carbon compound. During the energy-releasing phase, the phosphates are removed from both three-carbon compounds and used to produce four ATP molecules

Figure 5.12. The process of anaerobic respiration converts glucose into two lactate molecules in the absence of oxygen or within erythrocytes that lack mitochondria. During aerobic respiration, glucose is oxidized into two pyruvate molecules

Figure 5.13. Gluconeogenesis

Figure 5.14. Gluconeogenesis is the synthesis of glucose from pyruvate, lactate, glycerol, alanine, or glutamate

Figure 5.15. Glycolysis vs. gluconeogenesis

Figure 5.16. Glycogen metabolism

Figure 5.17. Glycogen

Figure 5.18. Complementary roles of insulin and glucagon

Figure 5.19. Insulin is a major regulator of metabolism and organ function

Figure 6.1. Overview of lipid metabolism

Figure 6.2. A triglyceride molecule (a) breaks down into a monoglyceride (b)

Figure 6.3. Classification of lipids

Figure 6.4. Fatty acids

Figure 6.5. The chemical structure of a triglyceride, showing the glycerol backbone and three attached fatty acids

Figure 6.6. A phospholipid molecule consists of a polar phosphate "head," which is hydrophilic, and a non-polar lipid "tail," which is hydrophobic

Figure 6.7. Lipid digestion and absorption

Figure 6.8. Bile salt

Figure 6.9. Digestion begins in the mouth and continues as food travels through the small intestine. Most absorption occurs in the small intestine

Figure 6.10. Overview of lipoprotein functions in the body

Figure 6.11. Chylomicrons contain triglycerides, cholesterol molecules, and other apolipoproteins (protein molecules). They function to carry these water-insoluble molecules from the intestine, through

the lymphatic system, and into the bloodstream, which carries the lipids to adipose tissue for storage
Figure 6.12. Lymphatic system
Figure 6.13. Beta-oxidation of fatty acid
Figure 6.14. Activation of fatty acids through coenzyme A
Figure 6.15. Carnitine shuttles fatty acids into the mitochondria
Figure 6.16. Lipids may follow one of several pathways during metabolism. Glycerol and fatty acids follow different pathways
Figure 6.17. Schematic of key steps in lipogenesis: acetyl-CoA is carboxylated by acetyl-CoA carboxylase (ACC) to form malonyl-CoA. In the rate-limiting step, malonyl-CoA is synthesized into palmitic acid and various other fatty acids via fatty acid synthase (FASN). These fatty acids are accumulated and stored as lipid droplets, which can be used as a fuel source in proliferating tumor cells
Figure 6.18. Dysregulation of lipid metabolism can confer metabolic disorders and trigger cancer
Figure 6.19. Hyperlipidemia
Figure 6.20. Fatty liver disease
Figure 6.21. Metabolic syndrome
Figure 7.1. Enzymes in the stomach and small intestine break down proteins into amino acids. HCl in the stomach aids in proteolysis, and hormones secreted by intestinal cells direct the digestive processes
Figure 7.2. Amino acid metabolism
Figure 7.3. Types of protein structure
Figure 7.4. General structure of an amino acid
Figure 7.5. Levels of protein structure
Figure 7.6. Protein before and after folding
Figure 7.7. Digestion of proteins
Figure 7.8. Protein digestion in the human GI tract
Figure 7.9. Enzymatic digestion of proteins begins in the stomach with the action of the enzyme pepsin
Figure 7.10. Overview of amino acid metabolism
Figure 7.11. Transamination and deamination processes
Figure 7.12. Nutrients follow a complex pathway from ingestion through anabolism and catabolism to energy production
Figure 7.13. Protein synthesis
Figure 7.14. Transcription and translation process of protein synthesis
Figure 7.15. Ribosomes interact with mRNA to produce proteins in a process called translation
Figure 7.16. Post-translational modifications
Figure 7.17. Regulation of protein synthesis and degradation pathways
Figure 7.18. Active older adults jogging outdoors, representing healthy aging and wellness
Figure 7.19. Protein metabolism disorder
Figure 7.20. Inborn errors of metabolism
Figure 7.21. Protein-energy malnutrition: (A) kwashiorkor; and (B) marasmus

Figure 7.22. Effects of excessive protein intake on the body
Figure 8.1. 3D illustration of a DNA double helix structure
Figure 8.2. Nucleotide
Figure 8.3. Structure of nucleotides
Figure 8.4. A nucleotide is made up of three components: A nitrogenous base, a pentose sugar, and a phosphate group
Figure 8.5. The nitrogenous bases found in DNA and RNA
Figure 8.6. The *de novo* pyrimidine and purine synthesis pathways. (A) Schematic of the *de novo* pyrimidine synthesis pathway; and (B) schematic of the *de novo* and purine salvage pathways
Figure 8.7. *De novo* nucleotide synthesis
Figure 8.8. Salvage pathway
Figure 8.9. Human purine metabolism. Pertinent pathways: Formation of the purine nucleotide inosine monophosphate (IMP) from non-purine precursors (synthesis *de novo*), or purine bases (salvage reactions); purine nucleotide interconversion reactions; degradation to the end product uric acid (catabolic reactions)
Figure 8.10. The degradation of purine nucleotides to uric acid, illustrating some of the genetic diseases associated with this pathway
Figure 8.11. Tophaceous gout
Figure 8.12. Pyrimidine metabolism
Figure 8.13. Pyrimidine metabolism pathways: synthesis and degradation
Figure 8.14. Disorders of pyrimidine metabolism
Figure 8.15. Nucleoside diphosphate kinases
Figure 8.16. Schematic showing the structure of nucleoside triphosphates
Figure 8.17. Diseases of nucleotide metabolism
Figure 8.18. Interactions between nucleotide metabolism and host immunity. Cancer cells could release metabolites from nucleotide metabolism, such as ATP, adenosine to (A) regulate immunoregulatory cells through adenosine and purinergic receptors; (B) in cancer cells, disrupted nucleotide pool could raise tumor immunogenicity; and (C) microbes release nucleoside analogs to regulate immunity
Figure 8.19. Current and potential targets for therapeutic interventions of diabetic kidney disease (DKD)
Figure 9.1. B vitamins coenzyme roles
Figure 9.2. Vitamins
Figure 9.3. A cofactor is a non-protein chemical compound that is required for the protein's biological activity. Many enzymes require cofactors to function properly
Figure 9.4. Types of vitamins
Figure 9.5. Water-soluble vitamins
Figure 9.6. Fat-soluble vitamins
Figure 9.7. A diagram illustrating the roles of various vitamins in different organ systems
Figure 9.8. Assorted dietary supplements and coenzyme-rich capsules
Figure 9.9. Coenzyme A

Figure 9.10. Sources of vitamins

Figure 9.11. Assortment of nutrient-rich foods including seafood, legumes, fruits, and vegetables

Figure 9.12. Vitamin B2 (riboflavin)

Figure 9.13. Vitamins deficiency

Figure 9.14. Summary of causes of vitamin D deficiency and diseases and disorders associated with vitamin D deficiency

Figure 9.15. Symptoms of too much vitamin D

Figure 9.16. Conceptual image of a doctor interacting with digital health technology

Figure 9.17. A comprehensive review and recent advances of vitamin C: Overview, functions, sources, applications, market survey, and processes

Figure 9.18. Food scientist conducting laboratory testing on various food samples

Figure 10.1. Hormonal involvement in responses to a stimulus. A challenge to the integrity of the organism elicits a response that includes the release of one or more hormones. These hormones generate signals at or within target cells, and these signals regulate a variety of biological processes that provide for a coordinated response to the stimulus or challenge.

Figure 10.2. Hormones

Figure 10.3. Amine, peptide, protein, and steroid hormone structure

Figure 10.4. The structures of peptide hormones – (a) oxytocin; (b) growth hormone; and (c) follicle-stimulating hormone are shown. These peptide hormones are much larger than those derived from cholesterol or amino acids

Figure 10.5. 3D mesh model of the testosterone molecule

Figure 10.6. Mechanisms of hormone action

Figure 10.7. Signal transduction pathways

Figure 10.8. Ribbon diagram of the β_2-adrenergic receptor, a G protein-coupled receptor

Figure 10.9. VEGF receptors and ligands

Figure 10.10. Ion channel receptors

Figure 10.11. Insulin and glucagon regulate blood glucose levels

Figure 10.12. The thyroid system of the thyroid hormones T3 and T4

Figure 10.13. The renin-angiotensin-aldosterone system increases blood pressure and volume. The hormone ANP has antagonistic effects

Figure 10.14. Regulation of calcium homeostasis

Figure 10.15. Conceptual image representing hormonal imbalance with medical tools in the background

Figure 10.16. Diabetes mellitus

Figure 10.17. Hyperthyroidism and hypothyroidism

Figure 10.18. Cushing's syndrome

Figure 11.1. Molecular biology

Figure 11.2. Scientists conducting molecular biology research in a laboratory setting

Figure 11.3. DNA diagram representing the DNA structure
Figure 11.4. Double helix
Figure 11.5. Nucleotide composition and base pairing
Figure 11.6. Chromatin
Figure 11.7. DNA replication
Figure 11.8. DNA replication process
Figure 11.9. The enzymes of DNA replication
Figure 11.10. Gene expression
Figure 11.11. Ribosomes
Figure 11.12. Post-transcriptional modification
Figure 11.13. Molecular biology techniques
Figure 11.14. Polymerase chain reaction
Figure 11.15. Gel electrophoresis
Figure 11.16. Schematic overview of CRISPR-Cas9 gene editing. In the absence of a repair template, cells will repair the break via error-prone non-homologous end joining (NHEJ), leading to functional gene disruption (gene/protein knock-out). Alternatively, a repair template can be used to introduce specific sequence changes via homologous-directed repair (HDR)
Figure 11.17. Protein structure
Figure 11.18. Basic enzyme kinetics graphs
Figure 11.19. Applications of molecular biology
Figure 11.20. Genetic engineering
Figure 11.21. Personalized medicine
Figure 11.22. Innovation in agriculture
Figure 12.1. Genetic disorders
Figure 12.2. 3D illustration of human chromosomes
Figure 12.3. Types of genetic disorders
Figure 12.4. Single-gene disorders
Figure 12.5. Chromosomal abnormalities
Figure 12.6. The combination of environmental factors and genetic factors is the main culprit which takes responsible for causing multifactorial diseases
Figure 12.7. Mutations can lead to changes in the protein sequence encoded by the DNA
Figure 12.8. In the formation of gametes, it is equally likely that either one of a pair of alleles from one parent will be passed on to the offspring. This figure follows the possible combinations of alleles through two generations following a first-generation cross of homozygous dominant and homozygous recessive parents. The recessive phenotype, which is masked in the second generation, has a 1 in 4, or 25%, chance of reappearing in the third generation
Figure 12.9. Researchers analyzing genetic data through an interactive digital interface
Figure 12.10. Symptoms of Huntington's disease

Figure 12.11. Medical professional reviewing digital genomic data alongside a 3D DNA model
Figure 12.12. Genetic counseling
Figure 12.13. Treatment of genetic disorders
Figure 12.14. Genetic disease medical treatment
Figure 12.15. Gene therapy

PREFACE

Biochemistry serves as the bridge between the molecular world and the life processes that sustain health and disease. It examines the chemical foundations of living matter by studying the structure, function, and interactions of molecules within cells. The application of chemical principles to biological systems reveals how atoms and small compounds combine to form the large biomolecules essential for life. In doing so, it explains why energy transfer occurs in predictable ways, how information is coded and expressed, and how metabolic pathways maintain homeostasis in the face of ever-changing conditions. This science is indispensable for anyone seeking to understand how cells operate, how organs function together, and how perturbations at the molecular level can manifest as clinical disorders.

Over the past several decades, advances in analytical methods, ranging from spectrophotometry to mass spectrometry and from gene sequencing to biomarker assays, have significantly expanded our understanding of biochemical processes. Those developments have allowed researchers to track reaction mechanisms in real time, quantify trace molecules in complex fluids, and map out the pathways through which nutrients are assimilated, transformed, and excreted. As a result, our ability to diagnose disease, to monitor therapeutic interventions, and to develop targeted treatments has been greatly enhanced. Biochemistry thus provides the fundamental framework upon which modern medical diagnostics and therapeutics rest, and it equips practitioners with the insights needed to interpret laboratory results and design new strategies for health maintenance.

This volume, *Handbook of Medical Biochemistry, Volume 1: Foundations of Molecular and Metabolic Medicine,* offers a comprehensive survey of the chemical principles underlying human physiology and pathology. It is designed to serve both as an introductory guide for newcomers and as a detailed reference for seasoned professionals. By gathering contributions from leading researchers and clinicians, the text brings together established concepts and emerging trends in one coherent resource. Readers will find chapters that explain the basics of molecular interactions, explore the pathways that generate and utilize energy, and examine the biochemical basis of genetic and metabolic disorders.

Chapter 1 presents an overview of the field, tracing the history of biochemistry from early discoveries to current frontiers. It establishes the chemical language that underlies all subsequent chapters, defining key terms, describing the major classes of biomolecules, and explaining the experimental techniques used to study them. Chapter 2 focuses on biomolecules, detailing their chemical structures, physical properties, and roles in cellular architecture and function. It covers carbohydrates, lipids, proteins, and nucleic acids, emphasizing how their unique features enable their specific biological activities.

Chapter 3 examines enzymes, the molecular catalysts that accelerate virtually all chemical reactions in living systems. It explains enzyme kinetics, mechanisms of action, and factors that influence catalytic efficiency. The discussion extends to enzyme regulation, including allosteric control, covalent modification, and the impact of cofactors. Chapter 4 addresses bioenergetics, presenting the thermodynamic principles that govern the conversion of energy within cells. It describes how cells couple exergonic and endergonic reactions, the role of ATP as the universal energy currency, and the mechanisms of oxidative phosphorylation.

Chapter 5 is devoted to carbohydrate metabolism. It follows the pathways by which glucose is broken down for energy—glycolysis, the citric acid cycle, and the pentose phosphate pathway—and shows how these pathways interconnect with one another and with lipid and amino acid metabolism. Chapter 6 turns to lipid metabolism, charting the synthesis and degradation of fatty acids, the formation of triglycerides and phospholipids, and the regulation of lipid utilization in different tissues. This chapter also discusses the transport of lipids through the bloodstream and the role of lipoproteins in cardiovascular disease.

Chapter 7 explores protein and amino acid metabolism, covering protein turnover, the pathways of amino acid catabolism, and the mechanisms of nitrogen disposal. It describes the urea cycle, transamination reactions, and the biosynthesis of nonessential amino acids. Chapter 8 examines nucleotide metabolism, detailing the synthesis and degradation of purines and pyrimidines, the salvage pathways that recover bases and nucleosides, and the biochemical basis of disorders such as gout.

Chapter 9 addresses vitamins and coenzymes, small organic molecules that are indispensable for enzyme function. It explains their chemical structures, sources, and roles as carriers of chemical groups or electrons. Each vitamin is discussed in the context of its associated enzymes, the consequences of its deficiency, and its therapeutic applications. Chapter 10 covers hormones and signal transduction, showing how chemical signals are generated, released, and perceived by target cells. It presents the molecular mechanisms by which hormones exert their effects, including receptor binding, second-messenger systems, and gene regulation.

Chapter 11 surveys molecular biology, describing the biochemical processes involved in DNA replication, transcription, RNA processing, and translation. It highlights the interplay between proteins and nucleic acids, the regulation of gene expression, and the technologies—such as PCR and recombinant DNA methods—that have revolutionized both basic research and clinical diagnostics. Finally, Chapter 12 examines genetic disorders from a biochemical perspective, illustrating how mutations in genes can disrupt metabolic pathways and lead to disease. It offers case studies of inborn errors of metabolism, discusses the principles of newborn screening, and outlines emerging approaches to molecular therapy.

This handbook is intended for a diverse audience. Medical students will find clear explanations of concepts that underpin clinical laboratory tests and therapeutics. Graduate students in biochemistry or molecular biology will appreciate the depth of coverage and the integration of biochemical pathways with physiological contexts. Laboratory technicians and clinical chemists will benefit from practical insights into assay principles and the interpretation of results. Researchers seeking a reliable reference on metabolic pathways and enzyme mechanisms will also find this volume indispensable. Finally, this book aims to equip its readers with the knowledge needed to understand biochemical data, recognize the molecular basis of disease, and apply those insights in both research and clinical practice.